Essential Oils for Pain Relief

Essential Oil Recipes for
Pain Relief
for Diffusers, Roller Bottles,
Inhalers & more.

Rica V. Gadi

DISCLAIMER: This document is a compilation of recipe used successfully by EO enthusiasts who use onl high-quality, therapeutic-grade essential oils as determine by many factors including growth, growth locatior harvesting process, distillation method used, etc. Please b advised that not all essential oils are created equally, an not all essential oils are suitable for topical use or ingestior Please do your research before choosing the brand(s) essential oils you decide to use as well as supplies you use Always follow label directions on the essential oil bottles.

All the recipes in this book have been inspired by essentia oil believers. However, we are not medical practitioners an cannot diagnose, treat or prescribe treatment for an health condition or disease. Just a precaution, before usin any alternative medicines, natural supplements, c vitamins, you should always discuss the products you ar using or intend to use with your doctor, especially if you ar pregnant, trying to get pregnant or nursing.

All information contained within this book is for referenc purposes only, and is not intended to substitute advic given by a pharmacist, physician or other license health-care professional. As such, the author is nc responsible for any loss, claim or damage arising from us of the essential oil recipes contained herein.

This book is dedicated to all the strong people who are taking responsibility of your own well being and doing something to be better.

All my heartfelt gratitude to the following people: my mom Ruby Jane, you have made me everything I am today; my dad Nestor-- my eternal, my angel, and the source of my perseverance; Mommyling, my spiritual guide ; Ria & Joe, the true witnesses of my transformation and my foundation pillars; Ellie Jane, the sparkle of our eyes;

Juan, thanks for always encouraging me to push harder - you are my ONE; Rocco & Radha, my reason for everything.

The Love of my family and friends is the fountain of inspiration that never runs dry. Thank you for constantly inspiring me, motivating me, and loving me unconditionally.

This book will never be complete without the help of my trusted and talented friends the #NOWsuperstars and my #oilbularya friends

Blending Essential Oils to use for a very specific reason has become very popular in the recent years. There are several reasons why this is so. Blending EOs is basically about inhaling - as it has been proven that aromas have the ability to trigger feelings, emotions and personal memories.

With this in mind, it is obvious that everyone is unique when it comes to what triggers your senses. It all boils down to personal preference for the aroma to trigger what you want to unleash. Everyone is different and we all connect to the aroma differently so what might work for one might not work for another person.

Of course, we also want the blend we personalize to be therapeutic. This is the best reason why to blend essential oils. We want the blend we create to help us with a very specific emotion or physical condition. As much as smelling good is important in a blend, it is more important that we blend oils that is not only pleasing to the smell but also produces the therapeutic effect we are after.

Then you have to think about contraindications. Making sure the blend you create is safe to use.

I suggest that before blending find out if the oils you are using is safe for a condition you may have example, if you are pregnant, or have specific allergies. Consult your physician prior to moving forward.

The recipes I have in this book is a compilation of what has proven to work and favored by hundreds of EO enthusiasts. It takes out the guesswork to get you started.

Again, we urge you to read the recipes and make sure that this is safe for you to try.

The book is very specific to a physical and emotional condition. There are several recipes here because you might want to rotate and you may like one and not the other. There is also a variety of application. Some of us prefer to diffuse, some to make roller bottles, and others to create sprays.

I hope you enjoy this compilation, feel free to use the notes section and jot down your fave blends. There is a wonderful world of EO blending - this is just the beginning.

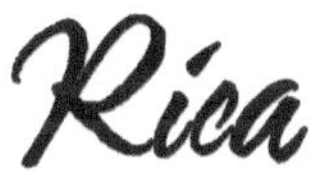

Table of Contents

Essential Oils For Pain Relief

Camphor: Camphor has an analgesic and anti-inflammatory components that work together to ease the pain and inflammation felt in all parts of the body. With the help of its sedative properties, it allows the body to relax and calm down letting the bruises, muscle aches and/or pains and arthritis heal faster.

Clove: Clove has an antiseptic property which is best in helping infected wounds throughout the body heal faster. It is commonly used to reduce pain and inflammation that is usually caused by headaches, swelling and joint muscle trauma. It also helps remove harmful toxins from that body that sometime can prevent proper healing to take place.

Eucalyptus Radiata: Eucalyptus Radiata essential oil comes from an evergreen tree native to Australia. It is part of the Myrtaceae plant family, and the leaves are steam distilled to product the essential oil. It is widely loved for its fresh, sharp, and clean aroma. Diffuse Eucalyptus Radiata oil to promote a stimulating and rejuvenating environment. There are many other uses for this essential oil, such as a key ingredient for an invigorating massage after activity.

Ginger: Ginger has anti-inflammatory properties that works together with the anti-nausea properties it contains to help reduce the pain and inflammation that can occur in the stomach. It also helps reduce inflammation that are caused by headaches, colds, muscle strains and arthritis.

Juniper: Juniper helps remove toxins that can cause the inflammation experienced. The properties it has help increase blood flow and circulation allowing the white blood cells to get to the affected area to gain faster healing. Juniper also help relax injured muscles in order to prevent further inflammation in the body.

Lavender: Lavender has a therapeutic property that is a great help in relieving inflammation. It helps the body to relax in order to reduce pain and inflammation on affected areas. It also has the properties that helps calm skin disorders such as psoriasis or eczema.

Peppermint: Peppermint has properties that helps relieve inflammation. It has pain reducing properties that helps reduce stiffness. It also reduce redness and cools the affected area.

Rose: Rose is great in helping relieve inflammation that is associated with many health problems. It helps reduce inflammation that is associated with depression, stress, fevers and muscle spasm. It helps reduce the pain felt because of the inflammation.

Rosemary: Rosemary is great for helping reduce blood inflammation at the same time increases blood flow and circulation to help with the healing process. It has anti-inflammatory properties that helps treat muscle pain as well as rheumatism.

Sweet Marjoram: Sweet marjoram has properties that make it a beneficial essential oil to use when helping to reduce inflammation. It helps reduce pain associated with inflammation caused by muscle injury and arthritis. It also has sedative properties that are important in the healing process our body does.

Yarrow: Yarrow helps in blood flow and circulation that relieves inflammation that is associated with arthritis. It helps reduce inflammation in areas like the digestive and respiratory system. It also helps promote healing and in the removal of harmful toxins in

our body which slow down the healing process

The Blending Process

These EOs are categorized by aromas, and EOs from the same group usually blend fantastically together.

- Floral – Lavender, Geranium, Jasmine
- Woodsy – Pine, Cedarwood
- Earthy – Vetiver, Patchouli
- Herbaceous – Marjoram, Rosemary, Basil
- Minty – Peppermint, Spearmint, Wintergreen
- Medicinal – Eucalyptus, Frankincense, Melaleuca
- Spicy – Pepper, Clove, Cinnamon
- Oriental – Ginger, Patchouli
- Citrus – Wild Orange, Lemon, Lime

Select oils that will give you with the health benefits you are looking to remedy. For increased energy choose: Grapefruit, Lemon, Orange, or Citrus. For Calming and Relaxation choose: Lavender, Cedarwood, or Chamomile. You are encouraged to experiment and play with your oils to see which blends work for you.

TIPS:

- Combine Floral EOs with Woodsy, Spicy and Citrus aromas
- Minty EOs with Woodsy, Earthy, Herbaceous and Citrus aromas
- Earthy EOs with Woodsy and Minty aromas
- Citrus EOs with Floral, Woodsy, Minty, Spicy and Oriental aromas

Diffuse

Diffusing Essential Oils is the safest method to enjoy Essential Oils without the risk of an allergic reaction.

Diffusing Essential Oils
Some Tidbits You Need To Know

Our sense of smell is one of our most powerful senses and as you have noticed in your own experience that some scents affect your more positively in your minds than others. The body contains over 1,000 receptor for smell—way more receptors than for any of our other senses.

Diffusion Essential Oils means the process vaporize oils into air by releasing tiny amounts into the air Inhalation is totally safe and is super low risk. Chances of any EO rising to dangerous levels while diffusion i slim to none.

Diffusing Essential Oils around newborns, babies young children, pregnant or nursing women, and pets should be done with caution. Read up on safety.

It is advisable that Diffusing Essential Oils for only about 15-30 minutes at a time to be most effective NEVER leave your diffuser on overnight. Make sure your diffuser is filled with the right amount of water and you understand the operating directions.

While diffusing essential oils, be sure that your space has great ventilation. Crack a window open if the scent become to strong.

Never add Carrier Oils to your diffuser. This may cause your diffuser to malfunction. Clean your diffuser at least 3 times a week with warm water and natural soap to ensure the diffuser is well maintained and bacteria and mold does not accumulate.

Diffusing Essential Oils Basic Guidelines

Just a few things you need to know and prepare before getting started Diffusing Essential Oils.

Things you need:
Ultrasonic Oil Diffuser
Essential Oils
Water

Just follow the number of drops in the recipe, drop on to an oil diffuser and fill the rest with water.

All diffusers are different and will have its own water minimum and maximum level. Read the diffuser instruction before use.

Ideally, it is best to diffuse for 15-30 minutes and turn off the diffuser. The effect should be good for at least 2-3 hours. Turn your diffuser back on after 3 hours to reinforce oil diffusing effects.

It is not advisable to use EO in humidifiers.

These are not made to release EOS

Diffuser Recipes

Here's a thought for you:

You may be wondering how aroma can simply eliminate physical pain. There's a simple answer to this : Pain whether coming from physical or emotion share the same space in our brains. Since emotions are closely connected to the sensory centers of the brain, what we feel emotionally can manifest, through pain we feel physically

So for here are a few recipes that can help you manage your emotions so it reduces the negative effects it may manifest in the physical body.

3 Drops Lavender
3 Drops Geranium
2 Drops Roman Chamomile
2 Drops Clary Sage
2 Drops Ylang Ylang

****

3 Drops Lavender
3 Drops Lime
3 Drops Mandarin

****

4 Drops Lavender
2 Drops Cedarwood
2 Drops Wild Orange
1 Drop Ylang Ylang

****

3 Drops Frankincense
2 Drops Copaiba

****

3 Drops Lavender
2 Drops Stress Away
2 Drops Frankincense

****

5 Drops Frankincense
5 Drops Stress Away

****

3 Drops Peppermint
5 Drops Lavender
2 Drops Stress Away

****

4 Drops Bergamont
5 Drops Frankincense

****

4 Drops Stress Away
4 Drops Orange

****

2 Drops Purification
3 Drops Lemon
3 Drops Orange

****

2 Drops Grapefruit
2 Drops Bergamot
2 Drops Lime

2 Drops Ginger
1 Drop Sandalwood

****

3 Drops Orange
3 Drops Patchouli

****

2 Drops Lavender
2 Drops Cedarwood
2 Drops Roman Chamomile

****

4 Drops Lavender
3 Drops Geranium
2 Drops Roman Chamomile
2 Drops Clary Sage
2 Drops Ylang Ylang

****

4 Drops Lavender
3 Drops Chamomile

****

2 Drops Vetiver
2 Drops Cedarwood

****

2 Drops Grounding Blend
2 Drops Lavender

****

1 Drop Lavender
1 Drop Sweet (Wild) Orange
1 Drop Cedarwood
1 Drop Frankincense

****

2 Drops Lavender
2 Drops Lime
1 Drop Spearmint

****

2 Drops Lavender
2 Drops Bergamot
1 Drop Frankincense

****

2 Drops Juniper Berry
2 Drops Orange
1 Drop Lemon
1 Drop White Fir

****

2 Drops Eucalyptus
2 Drops Geranium
1 Drop Lemon
1 Drop Thyme

****

1 Drops Roman Chamomile
3 Drops Lavender
4 Drops Sandalwood
3 Drops Lemon

****

5 Drops Lavender
2 Drops Cedarwood
2 Drops Vetiver
2 Drops Patchouli

****

3 Drops Orange
2 Drops Lemon
1 Drop Peppermint

****

3 Drops Rosemary
2 Drops Peppermint
1 Drop Basil

****

2 Drops Sandalwood
2 Drops Frankincense
2 Drops Bergamot

****

4 Drops Peppermint
3 Drops Geranium

****

3 Drops Eucalyptus
3 Drops Rosemary

****

3 Drops White Fir
3 Drops Orange

Bonus Diffuser Recipes

Ultimate R & R
2 Drops Copaiba
4 Drops Lavender

Cares Away
5 Drops Lavender
3 Drops Lemongrass

Soothe Balm
4 Drops M-grain
2 Drops Peppermint
2 Drops Lavender

Mind Meditation
3 Drops Patchouli
3 Drops Ylang Ylang

Taming the Storm
2 Drops Lavender
2 Drops Cedarwood
2 Drops Vetiver

After Hours Special
3 Drops Peppermint
3 Drops Lime

Roll

Essential Oil Roller Bottles is the easiest method to enjoy Essential Oils Anywhere and Whenever.

Blending Essential Oils in a Roller Bottle
Some Tidbits You Need To Know

Essential Oils are usually super concentrated and too hard to measure how much to actually put straight from the bottle.

Roller bottles are a way that you are able to create blends ready to use with the right dilution. It allows your EO to last longer.

It also makes it easier to apply exactly where you want to target without getting it all over the place.

It is handy and easy to carry in your purse ready to use at any time you want to.

I like to apply EOs at the bottom of the feet for many reasons. Our feet have bigger pores than any other skin in our bodies. this means that they are able to suck in the therapeutic compounds in our blend into the bloodstream faster that any other part of the body. Imagine comparing a normal straw to an oversized straw and how much more you can suck in with the latter. This is how the soles of our feet is compared to the rest of the skin in our bodies.

The skin on our feet is also less sensitive and is designed to withstand some abuse. The risk of having an irritation from EOS is less likely to happen when applied on the feet.

The feet don't have the glands that act as a barrier. Sebaceous glands are glands in our skin that produces an oily substance called Sebum, for the purpose of lubricating and waterproofing the skin. Since this is oil and if you put oil on top of oil, it can act as a barrier or it may slow down penetration.

The feet and palms of our hands are the only skin that don't have these, so it is ideal to apply Essential Oils to the feet for maximum penetration.

Now, it would be hard to apply oils directly and very mess, right? Roller bottles make it super easy and convenient to roll the EOs at the bottom of our feet.

Carrier Oils Info

Carrier oils are vegetable-based oils with their own healing properties that dilute essential oils used to help carry the EOs into the skin.

Essential oils are highly concentrated and could evaporate very quickly. The carrier oil is mixed with the essential oil so it could penetrate the skin before it actually evaporates. Although EOs are oils, it is actually not that oily. When mixed with a carrier oil, it allows you to have more of the essential oil into your skin without wasting EOS to evaporate, making the healing properties of the EO strong and more effective.

There are also Essential oils that are too strong to apply directly to the skin and may cause damage, so it is important to dilute them with a carrier oil.

Never add Carrier Oils to your diffuser. This may cause your diffuser to malfunction. Clean your diffuser at least 3 times a week with warm water and natural soap to ensure the diffuser is well maintained and bacteria and mold does not accumulate.

Carrier Oils

There are a lot of different carrier oils that you can use with EOs to dilute them in a roller bottle.

To name a few :

Almond Oil - moisturizing and stays liquid at room temperature. Do not use if you are allergic to nuts.

Apricot Kernel Oil - moisturizing and suitable for sensitive skin or kids. It is super gentle on the skin.

Avocado Oil - moisturizing and suitable for sensitive and damaged skin. Perfect for skin problems.Can be mixed with other carrier oils

Castor Oil - with antibacterial, antiviral and antifungal properties, use topically to eliminate pain and relieve skin irritation.

Coconut Oil - its antibacterial, antiviral and antifungal properties it is the best and most versatile for skin care. The skin absorbs this very quickly. It solidifies in room temp and may still have a slight coconut oil aroma in it - but you can get a fractionated coconut oil to eliminate the 2 challenges above.

Grapeseed Oil - not just for cooking but also great for topical application on the skin.

Jojoba Oil - one of my faves for skin care blends. This oil is the closest to our natural oil our skin produces to it is absorbed easily without being oily. Also amazing for massage oil blends.

Olive Oil - this is the oil for herb type oils. mostly used for cooking but can also be applied to the skin but would need to be blended with a carrier oil that is mild and absorb well with the skin.

Rosehip Seed Oil - super good for deep moisturizing or skin irritations. This oil has a high content of antioxidants and helps remedy dry, scarred and wounded skin.

Recommended Roller Bottle Dilution Guide

RECOMMENDED ROLL-ON BOTTLE DILUTION AMOUNTS

5 ml (1/6 oz.) Roll-on Bottle = ~100 drops (1tsp.)
10 ml (1/3 oz.) Roll-on Bottle = ~200 drops (2 tsp.)
30 ml. (1 oz.) Roll-on Bottle = ~600 drops (6 tsp.)

Roll-on Size	5 ml	10 ml	30 ml	Add EO drops to roll-on, then fill with carrier oil.	
Essential Oil Drops	1	2	6	1%	Dilution Percentage
	2	4	12	2%	
	3	6	18	3%	
	5	10	30	5%	
	10	20	60	10%	
	20	40	120	20%	
	25	50	150	25%	
	50	100	300	50%	

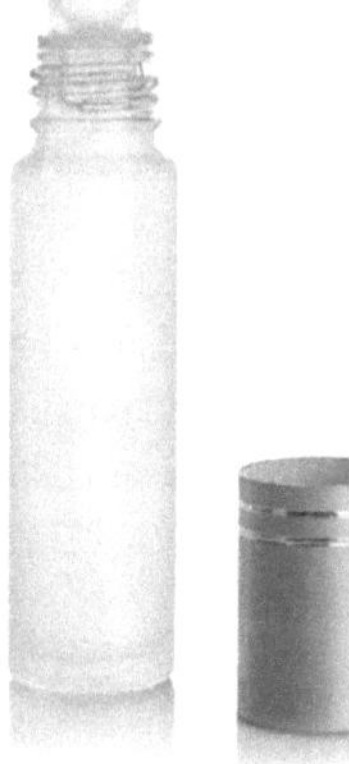

General Guidelines:
Birth to 12 months = .3-.5% dilution
1-5 years = 1.5-3% dilution
6-11 years = 1.5-5% dilution
12-17 years = 1.5-20% dilution
18 years and older = 1.5% dilution-Neat (no dilution)
Elderly or Sensitive Skin = 1-3% dilution
Daily Use = 2-5% dilution
Short Term Use = 10-25% dilution
Local Skin or Systemic Issues = 50% dilution-Neat

These are general guidelines suggestions--not absolute rules--based on traditional aromatheraphy practice.
(Kurt Schnaubelt PhD, Valerie Worwood, Robert Tisserand)

Dilution Basics:

How much you dilute your EO depends on different factors such as weight, sensitivity, health conditions EOs that are blended in or how long that blend has been used for. There is never an absolute dilution rule, it is you who knows about your level and tolerance. I feel that it is best to start with a higher dilution percentage and increase EO drops over time

To make sure your EO is safe, make sure that the oils you use are therapeutic grade and do your research on the source and extraction methods used to produce the oils.

Roller Bottle Blending Order

I normally just start with dropping the drops of oils into the **10mL roller bottle**, then adding the carrier o up until the shoulder of the bottle. Capping the bottl off with the roller and the bottle cap. Instead of shaking the bottle, i like to roll the bottle between m palms first for a minute or 2 for blending, then finishing it off with a few shakes.

NOTE: All recipes in this book is for a 10mL Roller Bottle. If you have a bigger or smaller roller bottle, adjust the number of EO drops based on the size of your bottle.

Roller Bottle Recipes

4 drops Frankincense
3 drops Lemongrass
2 drops Marjoram
4 drops Peppermint

****

4 drops Eucalyptus
4 drops Lavender
4 drops Deepblue

****

3 drops Clove
3 drops Black Pepper
5 drops Peppermint
5 drops Wintergreen

****

7 drops Peppermint
7 drops Lavender

****

3 drops Peppermint
2 drops Clove
3 drops Wintergreen
2 drops Black Pepper
2 drops Lemongrass

****

3 drops Valor or Valor II

3 drops wintergreen
3 drops Panaway
3 drops Copibia
3 drops of Relieve it

****

3 drops Wintergreen
3 drops Peppermint
2 drops Juniper
2 drops Lemongrass

****

5 drops Wintergreen
5 drops Valor
5 drops Peppermint
5 drops Panaway

****

5 drops Peppermint
5 drops Panaway
5 drops Valor
5 drops Wintergreen

****

6 drops Peppermint
2 drops Black Pepper
2 drops Clove

****

3 drops Wintergreen
3 drops Peppermint
2 drops Juniper Berry
2 drops Lemongrass

****

4 drops Marjoram
4 drops Lemongrass
4 drops Frankincense

****

6 drops Lavender
6 drops Melaleuca
6 drops Frankincense

****

2 drops Frankincense
2 drops Lavender
4 drops Cypress
1 drop Ginger
1 drop Peppermint

****

4 drops Lavender
4 drops Peppermint
2 drops Frankincense

****

5 drops Lavender

3 drops Peppermint
2 drops Eucalyptus

****

2 drops Lemon
2 drops Clove
2 drops Eucalyptus
2 drops Rosemary

****

4 drops Peppermint
2 drops Eucalyptus
2 drops Lemon
2 drops Rosemary

Bonus Recipes

Pain Relief Massage Oil Favorite

60mL Jojoba Oil (cold pressed)
8 drops Lavender
8 drops Peppermint
15 drops Frankincense

Pain Relief Massage Oil Secret

14 drops Frankincense
10 drops Sweet Orange
8 drops Turmeric
30mL Sweet Almond Oil

Pain Relief Bath Soak Blend

10 drops Frankincense
5 drops Lavender
5 drops Bergamot
1 cup Full-Cream/ Full-Fat Milk

Pain Relief Bath Salt Blend

1 cup Epsom Salt
¼ cup Dead Sea Salt
¼ cup Baking Soda
8-10 drops Essential Oils
(use any ingredient above or single oils)

Inhale

Essential Oil Inhalers are the most convenient way to enjoy Essential Oils Anywhere and Whenever.

Essential Oil Inhalers give you quick and easy access to the vast therapeutic benefits of essential oils.

Blending Essential Oils in an Inhaler
Some Tidbits You Need To Know

EO Inhalers or aroma sticks are compact tubes, with a cotton wick inside and a protective cover, to lock the aroma within.

Your preferred blend of essential oils is absorbed by the cotton wick, and safely enclosed in a tube that that fits inside of the cover. The cover is easily removed for access to the tube to breathe in the aroma. Usually lasts about 3 months, depending on the oil blend used.

I absolutely love these because they encourage me to take a moment during super stressful moments, and just breathe.

It is in times of stress when our breathing patterns often change and taking deep breaths promote a feeling of calm and inner peace. Breath work combined with visualization plus a relaxing inhaler, can offer relief to symptoms of stress and help your body to come back to the state of homeostasis.

Aroma Sticks can be carried in your tiny purse, even compact enough to fit in your pocket. You can enjoy your favorite EOs anywhere and you can use them with discretion.

I love diffusing, and do all the time but not everyone in my space may enjoy the scents I enjoy or they may not benefit from the therapeutic benefits of the EOs I am diffusing - so the inhaler is one way to not only enjoy my choice of blends but to keep in personal not affecting everyone else around me.

Inhalers not only benefits me but also keep those around me safe in case the oils I want to blend may pose a risk to those around me who may have health issue not advised to be exposed to my choice EOs/

When making Aroma Sticks, You may use your chosen EOs at 100% Concentration.

Inhaler Basic Guidelines

Breathe in slow and deep to absorb the EO molecules directly into your olfactory system.

Inhalers are super easy to use. You just remove the cap and inhale from the inhaler tube, count 1 to 5 slowly as you inhale. The EO molecules get drawn into our bloodstream through our nasal cavity and gets delivered throughout our entire body.

Simple to use, easy to cary, portable and compact. You never have to be without your favorite blends, ever.

Inhaler Blending Basics

Inhalers are super easy and simple to make.

All you need is an inhaler set which consist of the following:

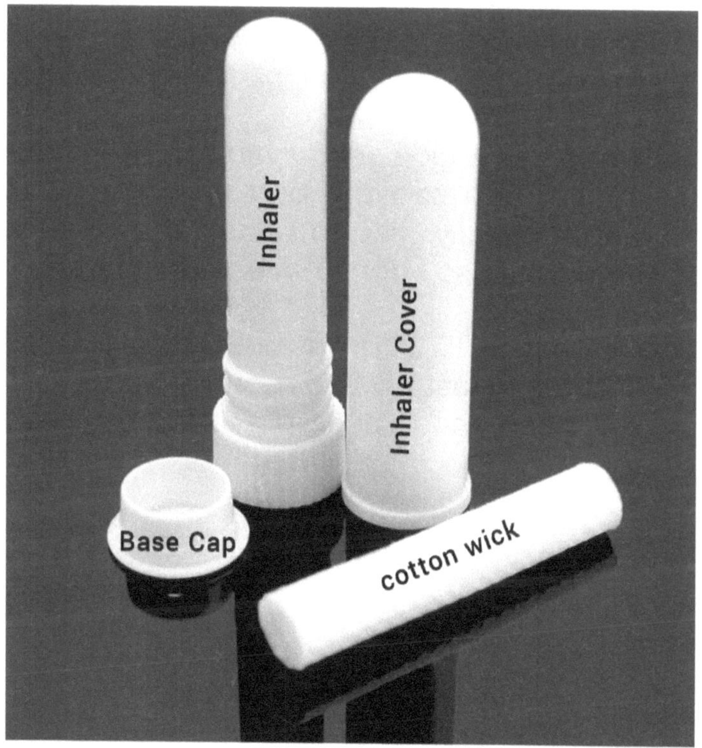

Inhaler, Inhaler Cover, Base Cap and Cotton Wick.

You will need your Essential Oils.

I like to use a pipette for precision and a small petri dish so I can see the oil.

Blending is super easy, just combine the drops and swirl it around in the petri dish and when you are satisfied you can go ahead and drop the cotton wick to absorb all the oil in the dish.

Once the wick is ready you can drop it in the inhaler and cap the bottom with the Base Cap. I usually like to secure the cover with the inhaler so I don't have to do it later.

I usually us 15-20 drops of EO total in a recipe and it can last up to 3 months. Some recipe will need more but on average it is in this range.

Inhaler Recipes

5 drops of Wild Orange
5 drops of Bergamot
5 drops of Sandalwood
5 drops of Ylang Ylang

****

7 drops of Vetiver
5 drops of Sandalwood or Cedarwood
4 drops of Ylang Ylang

****

4 drops of Ylang Ylang
7 drops of Orange
4 drops of Lavender

****

6 drops of Lemon
2 drops of Basil
2 drops of Rosemary
2 drops of Frankincense

****

6 drops of Lavender
3 drops of Lemon
3 drops of Ylang Ylang

****

3 Drops of Chamomile
6 Drops of Cedarwood or Sandalwood

3 Drops of Geranium
3 Drops of Bergamot
4 Drops of Lavender

****

10 drops of Roman Chamomile
5 drops of Lavender
3 drops of Vetiver

****

10 drops of Palmarosa
5 drops of Geranium
5 drops of Lavender

****

4 drops Lavender
4 drops Orange
4 drops Frankincense
3 drops Cedarwood

****

6 drops Lavender
5 drops Lime
4 drops Spearmint

****

8 drops of Lavender
4 drops of Roman Chamomile

****

6 drops of Geranium
6 drops of Rose
3 drops of Ylang Ylang

****

5 drops of Frankincense
4 drops of Ylang Ylang
3 drops of Sandalwood
3 drops of Patchouli

****

6 drops of Tangerine
4 drops of Juniper
3 drops of Bergamot
2 drops of Clary Sage

****

8 drops of Roman Chamomile
8 drops of Lavender
6 drops of Majoram
1 drop of Vetiver

****

6 drops of Peppermint
3 drops of Frankincense
3 drops of Lavender

3 drops of Chamomile

<u>Book Ordering</u>

To order your copy / copies of

Essential Oils for Pain Relief

please visit:
OilNaturalEmpress.com

You can also check out other titles available.

Bulk Pricing and
Affiliate Programs Available